Paul AND Me

*A Walk through
Parkinson's and Dementia*

JEAN WILLIAMS

ISBN 978-1-68570-058-4 (paperback)
ISBN 978-1-68570-059-1 (digital)

Christian Faith Publishing, Inc.
832 Park Avenue
Meadville, PA 16335
www.christianfaithpublishing.com

Printed in the United States of America

CONTENTS

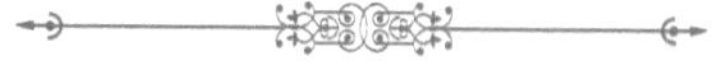

Preface..5

Chapter 1..7

   The Telephone Call..7
   The Diagnosis...8
   Missed Symptoms...10
   Parkinson's and Dementia Symptoms................12

Chapter 2..16

   Sisterly Duties...16
   The Ninety-Day Stay.......................................17
   Unexpected Family Drama..............................19
   Paul's Will..20
   Family and Staff Meetings...............................24

Chapter 3..25

   Manor Care, Second Stop, Rehabilitation.........25
   Shopping Spree..25
   Settling In...26
   Family Drama Continues.................................26

Chapter 4 28

    Money, Money, Money 28
    The Disappearance...29
    Third Move: Sunrise Assisted-Living Facility........29
    Hospital Visits..30
    The Falls 32

Chapter 5 34

    Down the Rabbit Hole: Juanita.............................34
    Court Filings..35
    Court Appearances...36

Chapter 6 39

    The Fourth and Final Move 39
    Hallucinations..40
    Hospice Care..40

Acknowledgments 43

PREFACE

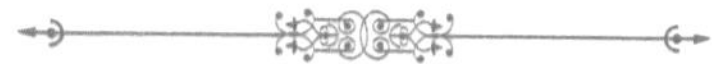

This is my first book. After guiding my brother through the twin diseases of dementia and Parkinson's until his death, I wanted to share my journey with others.

During my lifetime, I have been an educator, an administrative assistant, a tutor, a computer instructor, a wife, a mother, and a sister.

I was born in Washington, DC, and lived in a wonderful two-story red brick home with my parents and brothers and sisters. There were ten of us—six brothers and three sisters. I attended schools in Washington, DC, where I earned my bachelor's and master's degrees.

Now, I hope to add the word *author* to the story of my life.

CHAPTER 1

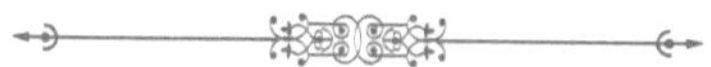

The Telephone Call

On a bright, sunny summer morning in 2010, while exercising in the morning sunlight in front of my picture window in Arlington, Virginia, I picked up the phone on the third ring. It was Paul, my older brother, who was one of six brothers. He, at the time, lived alone in the family home on Capitol Hill, Washington, DC. Since his last divorce, Paul, at seventy-eight years of age, lived by himself and took care of the debt-free two-story three-bedroom red brick home that our parents bought, paid for, and raised ten children in. He was retired—a federal employee—but for years worked a part-time job as a desk clerk.

I thought he was calling to see if I would pick him up and go out to breakfast with him at his favorite all-you-can-eat restaurant on Pennsylvania Avenue in Washington, DC. Often, when I thought of Paul, our family home, and Pennsylvania Avenue, I thought of all the parades I watched as a child in DC and the inaugural pageantry on Pennsylvania Avenue when new presidents were sworn in. I remember, after the swearing in, seeing Barack and Michelle Obama strolling down Pennsylvania Avenue, waving to the huge cheering crowds. Now, I am driving on Pennsylvania

Avenue to get Paul quickly to the hospital for a diagnosis and treatment.

Instead, I heard a familiar but shaky voice say, "Sis, I think I had a stroke, my arm hurts, and my hand is in a fist and won't open."

The smile faded fast from my face, as if I had been suddenly slapped. I considered calling an ambulance for him.

He said, "No, you come."

I immediately got dressed and drove in silence from Arlington, Virginia, across the Memorial Bridge, into Washington, DC. While driving across the Memorial Bridge, I observed the beautiful Lincoln Memorial, the Jefferson Memorial, and the Washington Monument. For a short period, I felt peaceful and stress-free.

When I saw him, I reassured him that everything was going to be fine. So off we went in my car to the Veterans Hospital in Washington, DC. Thus began our long, lonely, and life-changing chain of events into the world of dementia, Parkinson's, and family drama.

The Diagnosis

As we approached the hospital and saw the sign Veterans Hospital, I took a deep breath. I turned wearily into the parking area, and my car crept slowly up and down the parking lot aisles until I found a parking space. We looked at each other, and each of us simply stared but wordless before exiting the car and approaching the entrance. We showed our IDs as soon as we set foot inside the VA Hospital's doors and signed in at the security desk.

Once his name was called, I remained nearby during the preliminary intake interview. Paul sat quietly, very tense, fingers interlocked, and with a look of fear or foreboding on his face. While he was being examined, I worked the crossword puzzle in the *Washington Post* newspaper and then switched to working an easy sudoku puzzle on my tablet. After a while, I was asked to join him in the examination room. First, what seemed like good news became words that were not in my everyday vocabulary and would change us and our brother-sister relationship forever.

First, he had not had a stroke. He had fallen asleep in a chair while watching *The Tonight Show* on TV. His arm had been draped over the back of his comfortable chair, and somehow, the pressure on a nerve in the armpit caused the nerves in the arm and hand to contract.

Then, the doctor said to us, "Paul is probably in the early stages of dementia and Parkinson's. We need to further evaluate you, Paul."

We both were stunned. He sat silently in the examination cubicle. My mouth dropped open. I stared with my eyes wide in disbelief. Tears came to my eyes.

I said to the doctor, "Are you sure?"

My brother said nothing; he sat still, like he was frozen in time. Where was the person who usually talked about the latest TV episode, or the local or national news, or the answers to crossword puzzles, or the Ellery Queen novel that he was reading, or the latest jazz album that he recently bought? He didn't speak up at all. His face seemed devoid of expression.

We talked later as we drove back to his house. He asked me to go to the next appointment with him. I did. Paul and I had a vague idea of the effects of Parkinson's. The great boxer Mohammed Ali and the talented television actor Michael J. Fox both had Parkinson's diagnoses, which the media covered extensively.

I was more so in the dark concerning dementia. I had a general idea but not a real grasp of the effects of it. Also, I didn't know anyone with dementia. Now I do: my brother.

So another appointment was scheduled within a few weeks for him to see the neurologist. Of course, I planned to be by his side. I was. Thus, I started my monthly then weekly ritual of driving from Crystal City in Virginia to Capitol Hill in Washington, DC, to upper northwest Washington to the hospital.

Missed Symptoms

I was retired from teaching but kept busy tutoring young students in reading and math at a tutoring center in Bethesda two days a week. I was also teaching computer applications to adults on the weekend, after taking classes and becoming Microsoft certified.

Since I was divorced, my time was my own. Now, it seemed much of my time would now belong to Paul because of hospital visits and my desire to be supportive. Over the years, my other three sisters and three brothers had passed away, leaving me as the only remaining sister in the family.

I spent several days a month visiting him at home in DC because Abby, a brother who seemed very close to Paul at first, seemed to have simply stopped his brotherly visits and weekly phone calls. I wondered why. Paul either didn't seem to know why or wasn't going to say. Monthly, Paul and I had gone out to lunch, or he cooked us one of his favorite dishes. We ate, talked, watched TV, or worked on crossword puzzles. I saw no signs of anything wrong.

What is it I missed? Why did he seem so normal to me? Was I blind to the symptoms because he was my brother?

Then I recalled that he often shook his leg when sitting, he smiled but rarely laughed anymore, his writing was smaller, and he walked slower. I thought these were simply signs of aging.

One of the first things that he asked me to start doing was to pay his utility bills and taxes for the house he lived in—our family home. During that time, I thought everybody wrote checks to pay their bills, but not him. He gave me cash each month to purchase the money orders from the neighborhood Safeway store, which was about three blocks from his house. Twice a year, he paid the taxes on the house. Paul had a savings account, which he closely guarded. He took public transportation or a taxicab to his bank and took out cash monthly.

He did not have a checking account. So after paying his bills while at his house, I would open my laptop and read about dementia or Parkinson's while he watched TV.

I read a lot about Parkinson's and dementia before his next appointment, which was to see a neurologist. I was very anxious but tried not to show it.

We were there early. The preliminary diagnosis was correct.

At this point, my life became totally entwined with his. He was admitted and stayed for ninety long days. I visited four days a week, before or after work, every week for all the ninety days. I drove in from Virginia, across the Memorial Bridge, into Washington, DC to the Veterans Hospital.

The bridge seemed to get longer for each trip that I made. My heart ached for him during every mile I drove. I no longer had free time or quality time for me.

Parkinson's and Dementia Symptoms

This is what I learned about Parkinson's from the website National Parkinson Foundation:

10 Early Warning Signs of Parkinson's

- Stooping or Hunching Over
- Tremor or Shaking
- Small Handwriting
- Loss of Smell
- Trouble Sleeping
- Trouble Moving or Walking
- Soft or Low Voice
- Masked Face
- Dizziness or Fainting

Paul was experiencing at least four of these early warning signs.

It was also confirmed that he was in the early stages of dementia. Dementia is a brain problem resulting in memory loss, personality changes, and impaired intellectual functions.

He had a type of dementia called Lewy bodies. My brain is now in overload trying to absorb all this.

Dementia with Lewy Bodies (DLB)

Lewy bodies are microscopic deposits of a protein that form in some people's brains. They're named after the scientist who discovered them. The symptoms of DLB include:

- Problems thinking clearly, making decisions
- Memory problems
- Visual hallucinations
- Unusual sleepiness during the day
- Periods of "blanking out" or staring
- Problems with movement, including trembling, slowness, and trouble walking
- Dreams where you act out physically, including talking, walking, and kicking (Reprinted from WebMD)

Common Signs and Symptoms of dementia include:

- Memory loss
- Impaired judgment
- Difficulties with abstract thinking
- Inappropriate behavior
- Loss of communication skills
- Disorientation to time and place
- Gait, motor, and balance problems
- Hallucinations, paranoia, agitation (Reprinted from HGHelpGuide.org.)

There are 5 Stages of Dementia

Stage 1: No Impairment
Stage one represents no impairment in a person's abilities. Loved ones who get a score of 0 have no significant memory problems, are fully oriented in time and place, have normal judgment, can function, and are fully able to take care of their personal needs.

Stage 2: Questionable Impairment
A score of 0.5 represents very slight impairments. Your loved one may have minor memory inconsistencies. They might struggle to solve challenging problems and have trouble with timing. However, they can still manage their own personal care without any help.

Stage 3: Mild Impairment
With a score of 1, your loved one is noticeably impaired in each area, but the changes are still mild. Short-term memory is suffering. They are starting to become disoriented.

Stage 4: Moderate Impairment
A score of 2 means that your relative is moderately impaired. They need help taking care of hygiene. They need to be accompanied to social activities or to do chores. There is more disorientation.

They get lost and struggle to understand time relationships. Short-term memory is seriously impaired, and it is difficult to remember anything or anyone new.

Stage 5: Severe Impairment
The fifth stage of dementia is the most severe. At this point, your loved one cannot function at all without help. They have experienced extreme memory loss. Additionally, they have no understanding of orientation in time or geography. It is almost impossible to go out and engage in everyday activities, even with assistance. Help is required for attending to personal needs.

(Reprinted from the Healthline website; written by Mary Ellis.)

I hope the above information was helpful to you. All the information from Paul's doctors and the Healthline website was very enlightening to me.

CHAPTER 2

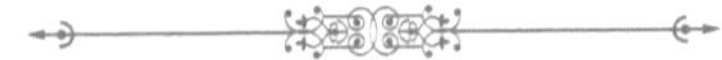

Sisterly Duties

After reading and learning about Parkinson's and dementia and meeting with his doctors and social workers, it was suggested that if Paul agreed, I should get two documents: a power of attorney and a health-care directive. Within a week, I saw an attorney and talked with him about the valid reasons for needing one. So I got the general POT. Paul signed it. I signed it. It was witnessed and notarized at the Veterans Hospital with Paul in person.

We left the hospital and went home for twenty-four hours so my darling brother could take care of some business. He had extra keys made for Elaine, our niece; Norman, our brother; and me to check weekly on the house, cut the grass, air out the house, clean out the refrigerator, trim the hedges, check the mail several times a week, and pay the monthly utilities.

How long would we have to do this? We all lived in separate residences. I lived in Virginia, Norman and Elaine in Maryland, and Paul in Washington, DC. This was not only our family home but also Paul's only home for the past twenty years. We had to do this for him, now that he seemed alone and confused.

That evening, something unusual happened that later would become a pattern. Our niece, Elaine, drove us to a KFC restaurant to get takeout before taking Paul back home. It would be his last night in his home on Capitol Hill in Washington, DC.

While she went in to place our order, Paul and I sat in the back of the car talking about his next appointment, which was to be tomorrow, and what to expect.

Suddenly, Paul said, "Don't turn around. Someone is looking at you in the window."

I was petrified but gradually felt compelled to look anyway. No one was there. Paul told me not to stare at the man. Only, no man was there or near the car. This was the beginning of knowing about his hallucinations.

The next day, we went back to the hospital. He was admitted.

The Ninety-Day Stay

Now, I realize that I am truly his support, his lifeline. I drove regularly from Arlington, Virginia, to Washington, DC, to help take care of the house, the yard and to the hospital to be the family member to consult with the doctors, the social worker, the dietician, and others.

One afternoon, I visited Paul and was startled. On his bed, his clothes were neatly folded. His toiletries were assembled next to his garment bag, and there he was quietly sitting expressionless in a chair in the corner of the room near a window. A health aide was getting ready to move him. I had not been notified.

I identified myself and asked, "Are you moving him? Are you releasing him? Is he going home?"

I was told "No release." He was being moved to the convalescence area of the hospital.

I said, "I am going too."

I did.

The next day, while visiting, Paul was examined and questioned by the attending physician. He was asked a series of end-of-life questions, which I heard while I was seated outside of the curtain. I heard Paul's responses too. Then the doctor asked him if he would repeat his answers in my presence. I was called to Paul's bedside; he was sitting up, lucid and ready to answer the questions with me being present. I held his hand; the doctor did assure him that these were routine questions and that he was not dying. The doctor explained the questions to Paul to make sure that he fully understood.

The questions were similar to these:

- If you could not breathe on your own, would you want a respirator, a machine to help you breathe?
- If you were unable to swallow or eat, would you want to be fed by artificial means, through a tube?
- If your heart stopped, would you want to be resuscitated?

He answered no to all the questions, and he and I signed off on the form the doctor had.

Later, I obtained a health-care directive on behalf of Paul. It was witnessed and signed by two people after he had signed it. This directive allowed medical personnel to inform me about his wishes concerning his health care. It allowed him to appoint or name me as an agent or person to be in charge of making health-care decisions for him if he became unable to make those decisions. It took effect when he could not communicate his medical wishes or became unable mentally or physically to do so.

During the ninety days that he was at the hospital, he had other medical issues. He had to have several blood transfusions and was experiencing hallucinations and mood swings. Through all this, Paul seemed himself most of the time, except for the family drama that had begun that I was unprepared for but had to deal with.

Unexpected Family Drama

During the time of his blood transfusions, he was in the critical care unit for three days and monitored twenty-four hours per day. His brother Abby, who had stopped visiting him while he was at home, suddenly started visiting at odd hours, usually near the end of visitation time or later. It seems that he stood over Paul's bed and remarked, "I told you that I would be the last man standing." Of course, Paul was not able to respond, but he probably heard his brother's words.

A nurse who was managing Paul's vital signs asked me what the term meant when I came to visit. I was shocked, as it obviously had meaning for this brother of mine. I gave the nurse a general meaning that the person uttering that phrase means to outlast, best, top anyone he is in competition with. Surely, there was no reason to be in competition with Paul who was seventy-eight years old, hospitalized, and in the critical care unit!

Things became even more bizarre when one day I drove to the house and had a snack, checked the mail, cut the grass, cleaned the windows on the lower lever, aired out the house, and trimmed the hedges. I finished trimming the hedges and was putting the clippings in the bag when Abby, our absentee brother, drove up, parked his car, walked over to me, and said, "Jean, you don't need to do this anymore because the house is between Paul and me."

I had no idea why this would be said to me when in the past five weeks he did nothing to keep the house from looking unlived in and had stopped visiting or calling Paul for the past year. I remarked that Elaine, our niece, and I had been doing this for over a year because Paul didn't feel up to it and was now hospitalized. Norman, another brother, also helped to keep the house clean and tidy and looking lived in.

Abby replied, "You have been informed," and left.

I had six brothers in all. Three were deceased. Abby was not being brotherly at all. Only meanness came across. Why? I didn't know.

Paul's Will

One day, my brother Norman and I visited Paul at the hospital. Abby was sitting there. When we entered the room, we could see a look of despair on Paul's face.

We said hello to Abby, gave Paul a kiss, and asked him, "What's the matter?"

He replied, "Ask him."

I did, and Abby said the most idiotic thing that I have ever heard: "Paul has a will. It needs to be turned upside down with a new executor."

I knew nothing about a will. I didn't know that he had enough money or property to even *think* about a will. He was part owner of the family home. He worked as a desk clerk for several apartment buildings since retiring and did not have a large pension.

I said to Abby, "How dare you? You can't tell Paul what to do concerning his will."

Brother Norman spoke in defense of Paul and said, "If he has money saved and has a will, it is his to do with as he pleases. You can't have a say so in what he does with it."

This angered Abby. He jumped up and threatened Norman, who is of slight build and stature. Abby had been a Golden Gloves boxer in his younger years. Norman, a senior, wore glasses, walked with a cane, and has had two hip-replacement surgeries. I was so worried about him being injured by Abby that I lunged between them. I, a senior, felt confident in preventing further trouble because I learned karate years ago—many years ago. I smile when I think of the possibility of me calling on a skill learned many years ago to keep the family peace.

I told Norman to leave and go wait for me in the car. Then I left the room and found the floor nurse. I explained what happened, and it seemed that Abby had been coming near the end of visiting time. Each time he left, Paul was agitated. So we agreed that after dinner, Paul would be seated outside his room, near the nursing station, not closed off in his room.

This was all so surreal because Abby owned his home outright and has a substantial pension. He has three grown daughters who are doing well financially. So why was he making a play for Paul's money, whatever the amount?

After Abby left, Paul said to me, "Sis, can you come early tomorrow so we can talk about my will?"

I asked no questions at this time and agreed to come early. When I arrived the next morning, Paul and I had a long talk after he ate breakfast and had his coffee. He told me that he had saved, over twenty years, almost $78,000. In his will, he had left $15,000 each for Abby, Norman, and me and $10,000 for our niece, who was also the executor. The remainder of his money was to be divided among Abby's four adult children.

It seems that according to Paul, when we had our private conversation, Abby saw his bank statement once when he came to pick Paul up to go out to lunch. He then tried unsuccessfully to get Paul to add his name to his personal savings account. Paul refused. He said, after all, that he always handled his own business, took care of the house, paid the real estate taxes, patched the roof, and cooked and cleaned for himself, so he saw no reason to add anyone's name to his account. Now, he knows that he made the right decision.

Now, I am confused and hurt at the very thought that my brother would want to cut other family members out of a will and have it all to himself when this was not money of his in any way. Suddenly, it seems that his brothers and sisters and niece didn't matter, nor did it matter that we all owned our own homes, were not in need, and were seniors with good incomes. Where was the family peace and compassion and wisdom that come with age? It seems to have eluded Abby.

Paul and I had been informed that what he had saved would have to go toward taking care of him. He realized now that all the money would probably be needed for his care since he has dementia and Parkinson's. He wanted me to handle his financial affairs since he could not return home. He spoke with the social worker and doctor alone and requested that he be allowed to leave the hospital the next day for four hours with me, and go to his bank to make it official that he would add my name to his account to pay for his hospital bills once he left the Veterans Hospital. He would have to spend down his money.

It was agreed and permitted. So we made plans to go to the bank after I went to his house and located one other form of ID that he had at home but didn't remember exactly where he kept. I needed to find his Social Security card, his voting ID card, or his government-issued ID to be used as a second ID. I had my driver's permit, my passport card, my voter registration card, and of course my power of attorney.

Before going to the bank, I called to see what was required. He and I both would need two pieces of identification. He forgot where he had put his other ID cards. He had with him his VA ID, which he had to have when he was admitted. Since my car was in the shop, Juanita, a distant cousin who called me occasionally, offered to drive me to Paul's house and help me search the house for Paul's ID. I actually met her during the funeral of Joseph, my older brother and her granddad. She was not the person I thought her to be when I accepted her help. I was too trusting because she was family. Big mistake on my part.

A few days before going to the bank, I needed to get linked into the Veterans Hospital computer system with Paul so that legally I could be informed of Paul's medical conditions, medications, and appointments—per his wishes. I went to the office to supply all my identifying information as next of kin as well as that of my brother Norman, in case I become ill and couldn't function on Paul's behalf.

Juanita became quite insistent that her name be added also. No, it couldn't happen. Two family-member names were all that was required to be entered into the computer system. It didn't happen. Mine and Norman's information was all that was required.

Why did she think for a minute that her name should be linked to my brother's personal information? Why? I found it perplexing.

Family and Staff Meetings

There were several staff meetings with Paul and family members in attendance. Those family members were Norman, Abby, and me. The staff informed us as to their interaction with Paul, his medical conditions, and their recommendations. The staff members were his attending physician, a registered nurse, the social worker, the physical therapist, and a dietician.

Then finally, during the third meeting, the attending physician told us that Paul definitely would not be going back home. Also, there wasn't bed space any longer for him at the VA Hospital. The beds were for the wounded vets returning home from war—mainly the Gulf, Iraq, and Afghanistan wars. Some were injured physically, some emotionally, some mentally. We were told that it was time to locate a community nursing facility for rehabilitation efforts first.

My brother Albert protested because he had a stroke, recovered, and was living in his own home. He was reminded that Paul had dementia and Parkinson's and that despite rehabilitation efforts he would soon require our twenty-four-hour care. There would be no making him better, no cure.

Therefore, the decision was made with me along with my brother Norman, the doctor, and the social worker to select a facility. We did. It was called Manor Care, which was located in Maryland.

CHAPTER 3

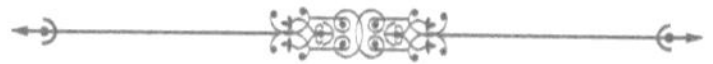

Manor Care, Second Stop, Rehabilitation

Moving to a rehabilitation or nursing facility didn't go without controversy because Albert (Abby) didn't agree and voiced his disagreement loudly. He wanted Paul to go elsewhere, but the social worker, Norman, and I were in agreement.

So on a sunny morning in May 2010, Paul, his belongings, and me left the Veterans Hospital and traveled by van to Paul's new home—Manor Care. Here, he would continue his rehab, which was covered by Medicare. This place was a good fit for Paul because his ex-wife resided there, and they had remained friends. They took meals together and enjoyed one another's company. She was very chatty and still loved Paul.

Shopping Spree

Elaine, my niece, and I went to Best Buy to purchase a thirty-seven-inch TV set for him. He loved watching comedy and law-and-order shows. We went to Target and purchased, at his request, a masculine bedspread, an extra pillow, and some 9.5 brown slippers. Also, later in the week, I purchased for him four short-sleeved shirts, three pairs of lightweight pants, and several pairs of underwear, socks, and pajamas. Also, I kept his mini fridge stocked with his favorite snacks and ice cream, which he shared with the ex-wife, Daphne, and now his constant companion at Manor Care.

Settling In

Paul seemed content in his new home. He knew that Abby would not visit him. Paul was lucky to be in a facility where he had a friend—his ex-wife, Daphne. They had dinner and dessert together. They watched TV together. They enjoyed having each other's company, again. I was happy for him. His life had some sort of normalcy now.

Family Drama Continues

Then one day, we went to Paul's house to get him a few more articles of personal clothing. Surprise! Abby had changed the locks on the house without informing or consulting with Paul or me. Paul, technically, is co-owner of the house with Abby. Abby, although executor of our dad's will, had never completed probate. So the deed was not changed to reflect that Paul and he were now the owners. My deceased parents were still the owners of the property.

My brother Abby believed that he would be the last man standing and would be the only owner of the property. The other family members either were deceased or were bought out of the property. Three of my siblings, heir to the family house, died within the last five years.

Now, I fully understand two mysterious comments that Abby had made earlier: one comment to me was that the house was between Paul and him, and the other to Paul, who was in the critical care unit at the time, that he, Abby, would be the last man standing.

27

CHAPTER 4

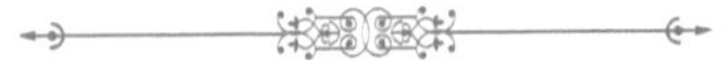

Money, Money, Money

Medicare payments for rehabilitation stopped after three months. I was not expecting this. I received a bill for part of the fourth month for $256 per day or $3,800. Now, I fully realize that Paul will need not only continuing care but also *costly* care. It's all about getting him the very best that his savings can provide for as long as possible. All his savings will definitely be needed to care for him. No family member now needs to be concerned about receiving any money as designated in his will. There will be no money left after paying for his care.

Elaine, on my behalf, contacted Abby by certified letter and requested that he arrange to buy Paul out of the family home. Abby could have used some of his savings, borrowed on his house, borrowed from his credit union, or allowed an investor to purchase Paul's share of the family house. At that time, the house was valued at $650,000. He would have easily recouped his payout, if he ever decided to complete probate.

Paul was still part owner of the house even though Al had never completed probate and both our parents were deceased. There was no reply from Abby at all. It didn't matter that Paul, who lived alone in the house for over twenty years, paid the taxes, made repairs, paid all utilities, kept all appliances in good working order, etc. If Paul could have gotten his part of the money, it would have gone to his continued care for dementia and Parkinson's once he had to be transferred to the nursing home.

The Disappearance

One evening, Paul was taken by ambulance to the hospital. He had fallen, and his blood pressure was quite elevated. Someone forgot to notify me. When there was a bed check, 10:30 p.m., Paul was unaccounted for. He couldn't be found. I was called and told that he was missing.

I was frantic, fearful and pictured him somewhere disoriented and afraid. I thought of the people whom I heard about on the news who had wandered away from home. Some were found safe, some were never found, and some were found dead.

As I was getting dressed to rush to Manor Care, I received the most precious phone call ever: my brother was safe. He was still at the hospital, still in the recovery room adjacent to the emergency room, sleeping. He was returned to Manor Care within the hour.

My heart returned to normal beating. My fears were subsided. Thank goodness!

Third Move: Sunrise Assisted-Living Facility

Paul's next stop is to a wonderful facility called Sunrise Assisted Living. In September 2010, Paul was transferred there. I was with him in body and spirit. He—standing tall, chatting with me—walked in totally unassisted. He walked a little slower and seemed resigned to his new placement. He was very impressed. He said it was like being in a hotel. It really was like that.

He was assigned his own room, which had a private shower; cable TV, which I made arrangements to pay for; and a large picture window, where he could watch the changing seasons. Breakfast, lunch, and dinner were served in a dining room with real china, real silverware, linen napkins, and menu listings for a full or mini meal. There were weekly hand massages and delightful musical presentations along with the expected rehabilitative exercises. Sometimes, Paul and I would have dinner in his room while watching TV or listening to jazz on his CD music changer, which I brought from home.

Hospital Visits

No time to think clearly anymore. A member of the staff called me early one morning to tell that Paul was rushed by ambulance, again, to the medical center. I met him there. He had extremely elevated blood pressure readings of cardiac enzymes; an x-ray showed a 1.5 nodular mass on the border of his heart as well as a renal mass on his kidney.

He was transferred to the stroke unit and remained there for four days. Elaine, Norman, and I visited him daily. He had an echocardiogram and further blood tests. I breathed a sigh of relief once his blood pressure returned to normal and the nodule was deemed noncancerous. After four days, he was returned by ambulance to Sunrise. So I'm expecting another $500 bill for ambulance services.

Then, as they say, life happened. Within six months, Parkinson's had begun to take its toll on his body. He lost muscle mass, and his muscles weakened. He had trouble walking unassisted. So he became wheelchair bound. After leaning too far forward, he fell from his wheelchair and was rushed to the Virginia Medical Center, which is one of the finest and best-rated hospitals in the state. The cost of the ambulance was over $500 round trip. Next, he became incontinent and had little control over his bladder. He could no longer shower, use the bathroom, or go to the dining room unassisted. The cost of his care per month increased as his condition worsened.

The increased cost did not include his medications for dementia, Parkinson's, and high blood pressure. I wrote monthly checks to a pharmacy in Richmond, Virginia, for $1,100 or more. After talking to another veteran at Sunrise about the high cost of medication, I was pleasantly enlightened that the Veterans Hospital would supply his medications because Paul had been initially treated there for all three conditions, and I had still kept up his monthly payments to the Veterans Hospital.

Over the next few months, I drove my brother to the Veterans Hospital for a few hours for the following reasons:

- To see his geriatric physician for a checkup.
- To apply for a supply of men's Depend. I had been buying them.
- To see his neurologist, again.
- To have the VA pharmacist check his medications.
- To apply to have the VA supply his medications.
- To visit the travel office to get them to provide Paul with transport to the VA Hospital.
- To see the ophthalmologist for his eye exam.
- To see the radiologist.

I continued to be with Paul through all his appointments. My regular visits to him, the medical appointments, and taking care of his finances were beginning to wear me down. I gave up my part-time job, tutoring. I had started to ignore my own health. But for now, Paul's care was first and foremost on my agenda.

The Falls

Paul fell out of his bed. He suffered minor pain and two small scratches. Nevertheless, he had to be sent by ambulance to the hospital for observation and treatment. He was released after four hours and returned to the facility. To solve this problem, his bed was lowered to be closer to the floor, and a rubber mat was placed beside his bed to prevent injury.

A week later, he fell again. This time, he was reaching for an invisible dog. He was hallucinating. Again an ambulance was called, and off he went to the hospital. I met him an hour later at the hospital. He experienced minor discomfort but no injuries. His blood pressure had spiked, so he was kept under observation and remained hospitalized for ten hours.

A third fall occurred a month later. He tried to quickly stand up and toppled over. Off to the hospital he was sent, again. He was having major hallucinations. The doctor examined him and asked him what happened.

He gave the doctor three different versions of what happened. None were true. First, he talked about being attacked in a park by muggers. Second, he said he fell fighting off a knife attack on the way home from work. Third, he thought he was in the kitchen at home and he fell dodging flying glass.

No serious injury resulted from the fall, just a minor abrasion on his leg. After several hours, he was sent back to Sunrise.

CHAPTER 5

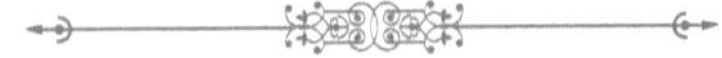

Down the Rabbit Hole: Juanita

When taking care of a loved one with money, beware! My relationship with this distant relative took a turn for the worse. She was not who she pretended to be. Now, I fully understood why this grandniece was trying to get her name attached to Paul's records while he was at the Veterans Hospital. He, like many other veterans, had elected not to get Part B of Medicare because they received all their care from the Veterans Hospital.

She called me late one night to chat about Paul and offered to fast-track his application for Part B of Medicare. I was grateful that she could help. She needed a copy of his medical records that indicated that he had dementia and Parkinson's and was wheelchair bound. So I drafted a letter requesting that she be given a copy of Paul's medical records for the sole purpose of securing Part B of Medicare on his behalf.

I called the assisted-living facility ahead of her visit and gave them the necessary identifying information for Paul and for me. I had gone to the Social Security office twice but couldn't endure the wait. I was number 35 the first time and number 27 the second time. I had to get to my job of teaching Microsoft computer classes. I had given up my tutoring part-time job, so I wanted to maintain some part of my life that was me. I had planned to go back in a couple of weeks to try again, so her suggestion was welcome.

Then three days later, I saw what was down the rabbit hole. It was Juanita. She was the proverbial snake in the grass. First, an assistant director called to tell me that she was there at the facility with another person attempting to question Paul about his care, his money, and me, as well as asking staff members about me and my visits to Paul. Why did she want that information from Paul? Who was the woman with her? Why didn't she ask me? I felt an unease that was beyond description. She was stopped and not allowed to question him, the staff, or any other residents about his care. She was told that she needed a court order.

Court Filings

Then within a few days, she dropped the other shoe. I received a letter from DC Superior Court informing me of court proceedings instituted by my great-niece Juanita Jackson against me. She had filed for guardianship of my brother and requested my removal from his financial life. My brother Norman also received the same letter from the court because he would become responsible for making decisions concerning Paul and his finances if I were unable to do so.

The day after receiving this notification of her intent, I found myself making my way into DC Superior Court to file a response to her petition. I was frightened. I was stunned. Later, I discovered that this occasionally happens when another family member finds that money is involved and they can possibly be named guardian and then have access to the money.

Court Appearances

Over the next four months, my brother Norman and I both received over fifteen petitions or notifications individually. I had to hire an attorney to represent me out of my own finances. The retainer was $7,500. My wonderful, caring niece, Angela, who lived in Philadelphia and was a retiree, also paid the initial $5,000. I was and am so grateful for her financial help. The first hearing was scheduled, and I had to file a response to the petition. I was surprised to be told that Paul would have a court-appointed attorney to represent him.

That attorney made an appointment with me. Before the hearing, his attorney interviewed me at home for two hours about my relationship with Paul and how I came to be his guardian and the circumstances that led up to his adding my name to his bank account. I had to produce six months of Paul's bank statements and my bank statements to show that there was no comingling of monies and that all money dispersed from his account for his care was accounted for. She corresponded with me several times during a span of eight months concerning Paul until the case was finalized.

She was satisfied after her interviews with me that I had been acting in good faith and in a trustworthy manner, that I was truly his guardian, and that any and all money dispensed from his savings was justified. Then I received a bill for $3,200 for her services.

Juanita, with her court filing, was legally allowed to go back to the assisted-living home with a geriatric health-care worker to question Paul about his care and my visits, as well as to interrogate the staff that interacted with him daily. Paul spoke highly of me and thankfully remembered that I visited many times a week, sometimes took meals with him, took him to all VA appointments, and often attended musical programs with him. The staff gave me high marks for my visits and interaction with him and for me taking care of his financial obligations every month and on time.

Finally, the day came when the judge would render his final decision as to whether Juanita would prevail and become my brother's guardian and have complete control over his bank account and his pension. If she did prevail, she would immediately be able to make all decisions concerning my brother. She would remove him from his current residence and take him home to a room in her home with a health-care worker. She would be in charge of the remainder of his bank account and pension. No money would be spent on twenty-four-hour care under a doctor's supervision. She would literally prevent me from visiting him.

Some important factors were the following:

- Paul expressed his wishes to the court that I remain his guardian.
- I had accompanied him to his numerous medical appointments.
- I visited him four to six times a week wherever he was being cared for.
- I accounted for and paid all his medical bills from his savings account.
- I had his power of attorney that he agreed to in the presence of witnesses.
- I, satisfactorily, supplied the court with all information or documents requested.
- I was retired and able to spend time with him; Juanita worked full-time and had a family.

The judge ruled that it was in the best interests of Paul that I remain his guardian and in charge of dispensing any and all money needed to care for him. We—Paul and I—won.

I had been too trusting of my family. This ordeal consumed hours and hours of my time with me reading and responding to the many petitions, appearing in court, meeting with my attorney and his attorney, obtaining and printing out six months of our bank statements, taking pictures of his former home to show that it was not wheelchair accessible and that the interior two-story house was not conducive for wheelchair functioning.

It was a victory that I cherished. It was worth it, though costly to me—a senior, a retiree, his sister.

CHAPTER 6

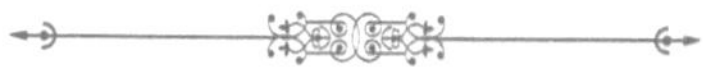

The Fourth and Final Move

After Paul had several falls from his bed or wheelchair, had an increasing numbers of hallucinations, and became totally incontinent, it was time for a nursing home. He needed twenty-four-hour care to meet his needs of bathing, dressing, shaving, feeding himself, and going to the bathroom with help.

So we made the move to a nursing home in Virginia, near my home. He had earlier mentioned donating his organs to medical science so that his brain and other organs could possibly help with understanding Parkinson's and dementia. That had been taken care of by me.

Within the space of two years, he lost muscle tone in his arms, hands, legs, and back. This is why he could no longer dress or feed himself at all. He had difficulty sitting upright in his wheelchair. He often leaned to one side of the wheel-chair. Since he was no longer able to sit stable in a regular wheelchair, he was put in a rolling reclining chair.

He was transferred to the next floor up, the fourth floor where mostly patients with dementia and Parkinson's were. He now was wheeled to the table where he sat with friends who simply now stared straight ahead expressionless as he often did, rarely spoke, needed to be fed, and, for the most part, just sat and didn't pay attention to the food that was placed in front of them, or the action or sound of the television, or any music that played.

He had friends who made him smile occasionally. One pal who made him smile was John. He shuffled into the dining room waving to all with one hand and holding up his pants with the other. He refused to wear a belt. Once in a while, John's pants would fall. He wore boxers. Everyone would laugh, while John would bow and say, "Thank you for being you." Another friend was Amy, who sat at another table and during lunch or dinner would burst into a Broadway song. She had a lovely voice. Some people would clap as she bowed or just stopped singing. Paul may or may not smile.

Hallucinations

It seemed, now, that this was the only time he spoke. The hallucinations had become his friends. He could see and hear them. He thought that he saw animals in the rooms, men dangling outside a plate glass window, and relatives on TV. He thought he saw our sister on TV and that he watched her walk out of the TV and sit at a table near him. He enjoyed seeing a former TV detective, Telly Savalas, sitting in the corner licking a lollipop. These were his friends who kept him content.

Hospice Care

Over time, the reclining chair with wheels was more like his daybed, something that allowed him to be out of his room for a few hours. He could no longer adjust his body himself to any position. He seemed to stop feeling anything. He could no longer sit, stand, communicate, or feed himself at all. Finally, he didn't understand the connection between the plate of food, his fingers, the utensils, and his mouth, so he needed to always be fed. Often, I would come and feed him at dinnertime.

Next came the realization that he could only swallow soft foods. He lost weight. My brother, who had weighed 160 pounds, now weighed only 110 pounds.

He started receiving—within the nursing home—hospice care, which meant that he met certain criteria for hospice care. He started receiving palliative care, not curative care. Paul

- had advanced dementia and Parkinson's;
- was not ambulatory, was wheelchair bound;
- was unable to bathe, dress, or feed himself;
- was totally incontinent;
- was unable to communicate effectively—limited speech;
- was unable to eat regular food—on a pureed diet; and
- had significant weight loss.

As of March 1, 2018, Paul was completely bedridden, and I visited him twice daily to give him a gentle back or shoulder rub, massage his hands with lotion, and try to give him water and sometimes just sit and hold his hands. I tried my best to be present often and to provide love and comfort.

Now, I have lost my brother and my friend. I lost his love, I lost his conversation, I lost his smile, I lost his self-assured walk, and I lost his strength. He lost too. He lost his memory, he lost his body muscle mass, he lost his communication skills, he lost his family, and he lost all world connections and his joy of life.

I quietly played for him, from my cell phone, a hymn, "Jesus, You Are the Center of My Joy." I quietly prayed not just for him but also for all the residents I met who had Parkinson's and dementia. There were many.

Did he know that I was there? I don't know if he heard or felt anything in his final days. He showed no recognition that he felt my presence when I touched him. He simply stared. He took in a miniscule amount of pureed food and water. In fact, the last week of his life, his mouth was sponged with water several times a day.

He, my brother, peacefully passed away on March 11, 2018, at 10:00 a.m., after a valiant eight-and-a-half-year fight with Parkinson's and dementia. Norman and I said our goodbyes to him. Our journey was now over. Paul's journey was over.

This was his sunset. I miss him greatly.

The End

ACKNOWLEDGMENTS

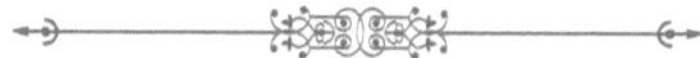

I wish to thank my brother Norman and my nieces Elaine and Angela for loving Paul unconditionally and for all their support and their time in walking this journey with me.

I wish to thank the VA Hospital, the assisted-living home, the nursing home, and hospice care for the excellent medical, physical, and emotional care and warm support that they all provided to my brother.

ABOUT THE AUTHOR

Jean William is a first-time writer. She was born in Washington, DC, and currently lives in Arlington, Virginia, with her husband. She received her master of arts degree from Trinity College. She is a retired teacher.